Prematurely Yours

Written and designed by

Kim Bryant R.N.   Becky Meloan R.N.

Prematurely Yours   319 Royal Drive   Bailey, CO 80421   800-767-0023

Fourth Printing 1999   Made in U.S.A.

ISBN 0-9614786-0-8

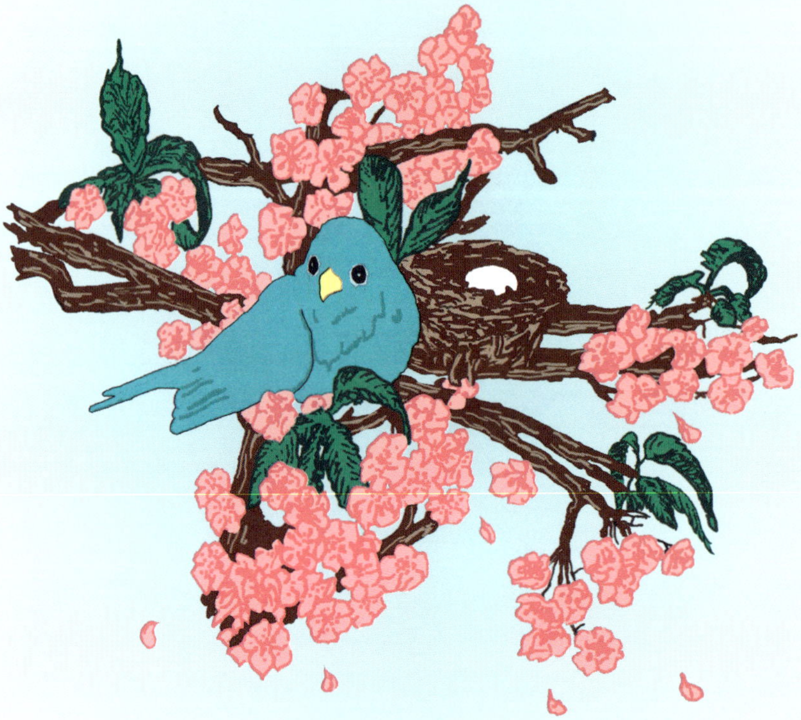

JAKOB MICHAEL HUDGINS

Baby's Name

WALNUT CREEK

Baby's Place of Birth

2-28-00	5:09 PM
Date	*Time*
2 lb 4 oz	13"
Weight	*Length*

How did you pick my name?

What does my name mean?

My nickname and why?

"JAKE"

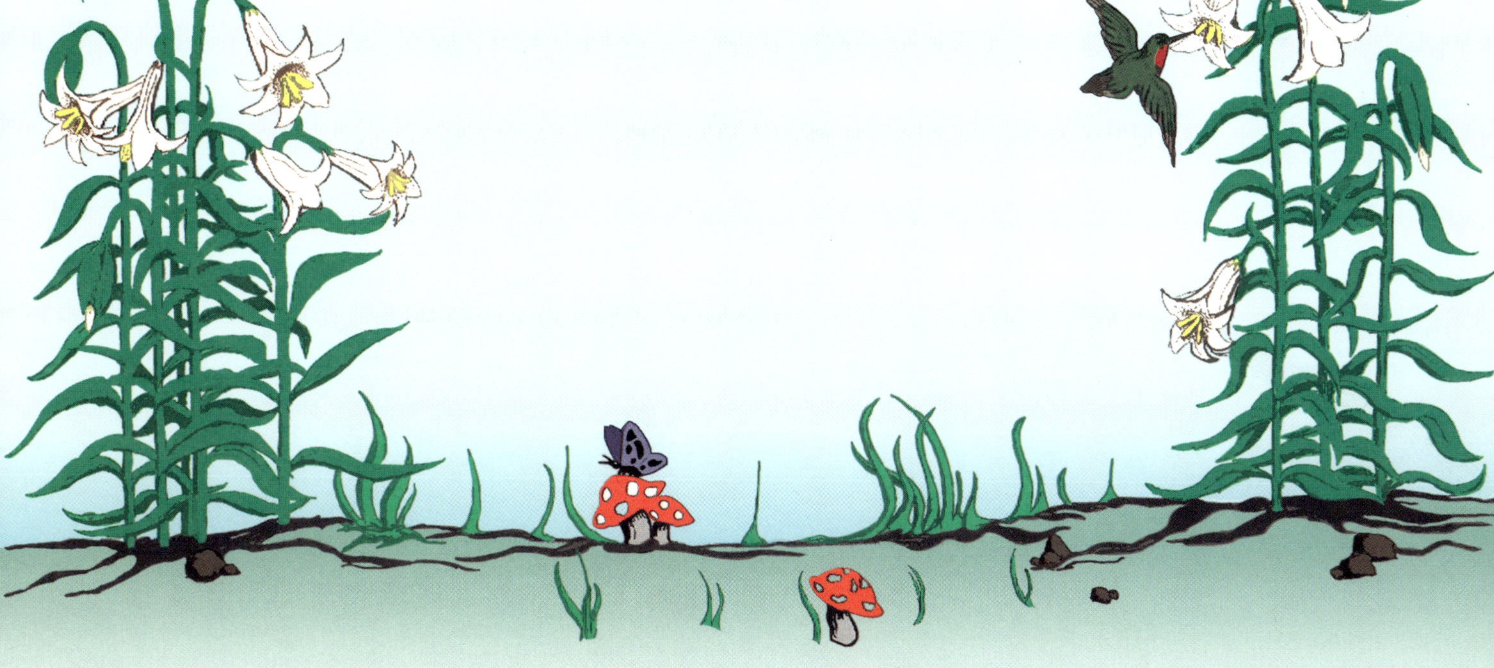

Your Comments About

The pregnancy

MOMMY TOLD ME ON MY BIRTHDAY THAT WE WERE GOING TO HAVE YOU

The labor

VERY Short ... 2 hrs 39 mins (2:30 p.m water broke ... 5:09 pm you were born)

The delivery

VERY FAST

Carol Candiotti, NP — *Mother's Doctor*

ZUKIN — *My Doctor*

My due date was MAY 28 *but I was born prematurely.*
date

My gestational age was 26 wks *weeks. My* APGAR *scores*

were ____________ *at one minute and* ____________ *at five minutes.*

Do you have any pictures of me before birth?

ultrasound picture

The World When I Was Born

CLINTON — *President*

GORÉ — *Vice-President*

ELIAN LITTLE BOY FROM CUBA

News

Actors

Actresses

SIXTH SENSE

Movies

TV Shows

FLY DIXIE CHICKS

CDs – Videos

EARL

Songs – Artists

BELL BOTTOM JEAN CAME BACK

Fads and Fashions

Sports Events

Sports Personalities

Baby's Identification

My Footprints

Hospital Bracelet

Lock of Hair

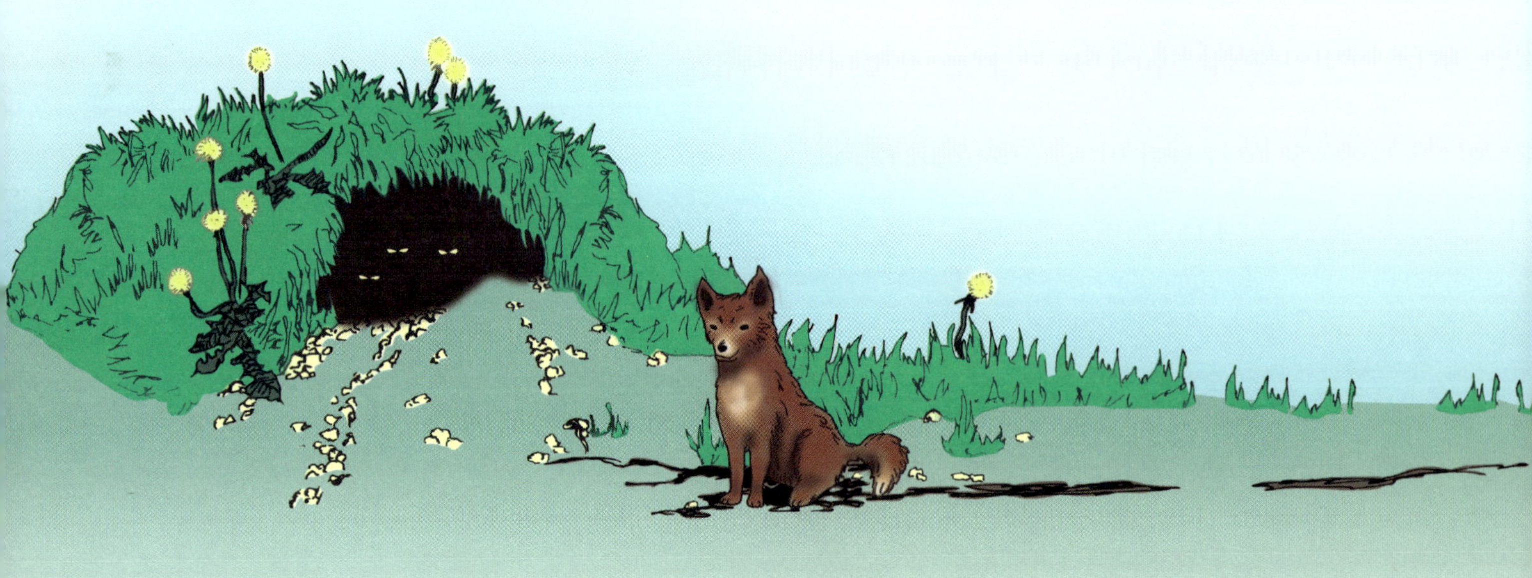

Baby's First Homes

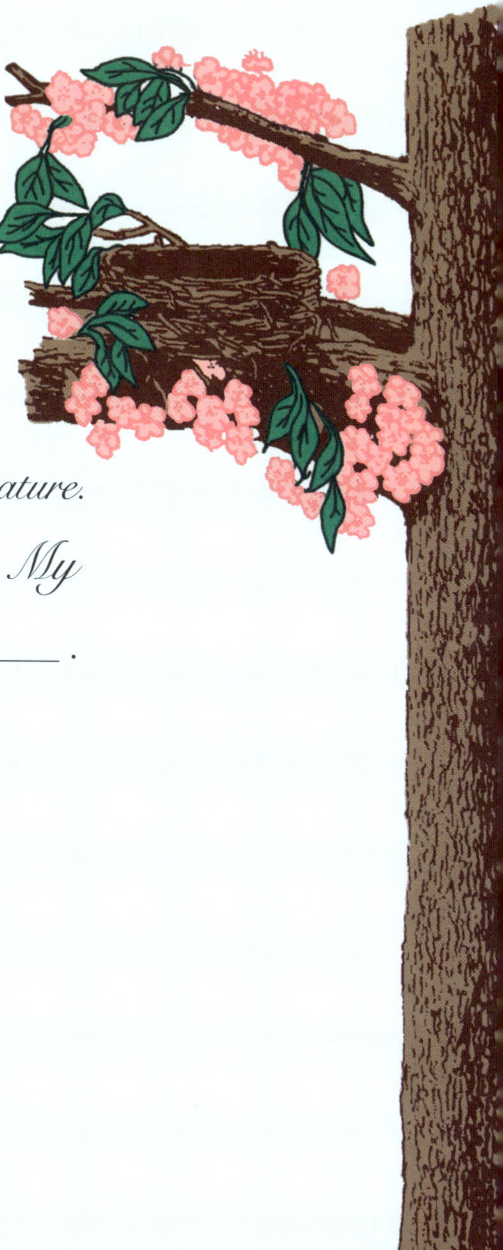

I started my life in the intensive care nursery on a warm bed called a radiant warmer. My parents first held me ____________________ .
date

When my condition improved, I moved into an isolette ____________________ . *My favorite house*
date

temperature started at ____________ *°C / °F.*

As I grew, I began to maintain my body temperature. I graduated to an open crib ____________________ . *My*
date

favorite crib toys were ________________________________ .

My parents first bathed me ____________________ .
date

Memorable neighbors in the nursery were

JESSICA

Your comments about my special care nursery

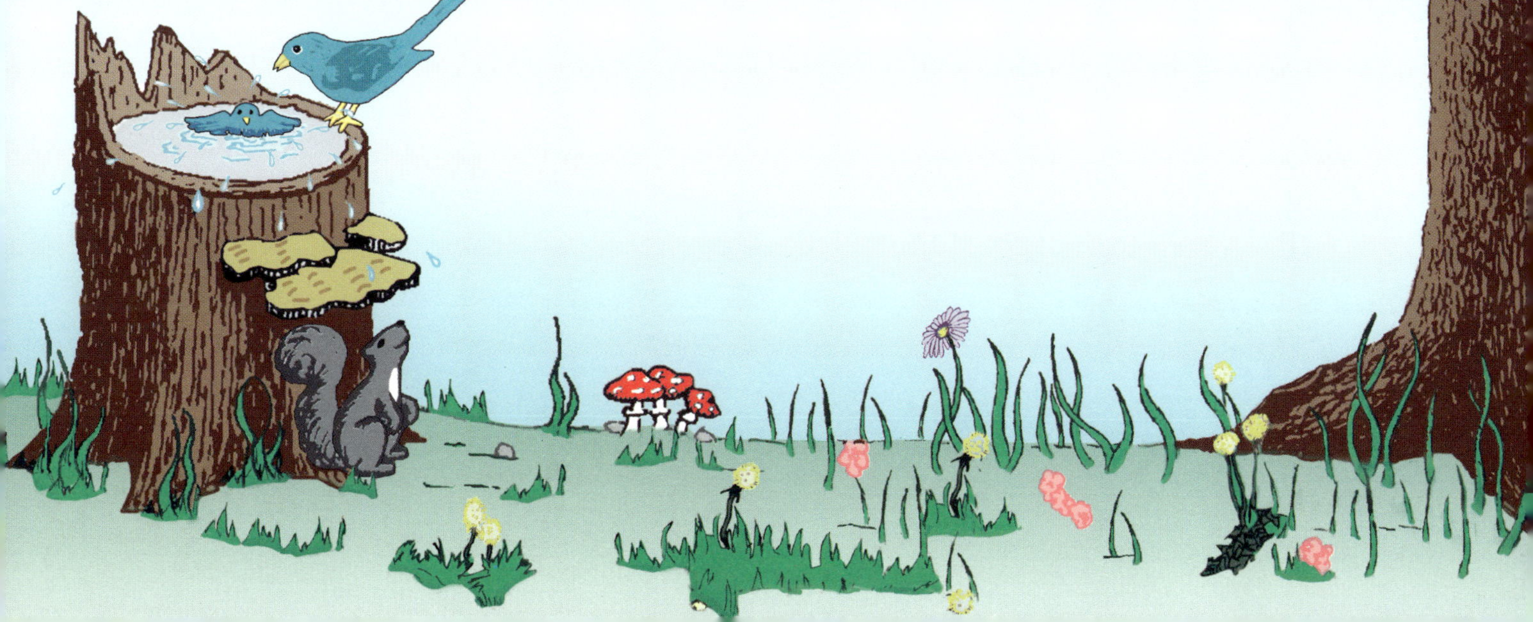

Because my lungs were immature, I needed extra help to breathe. I was

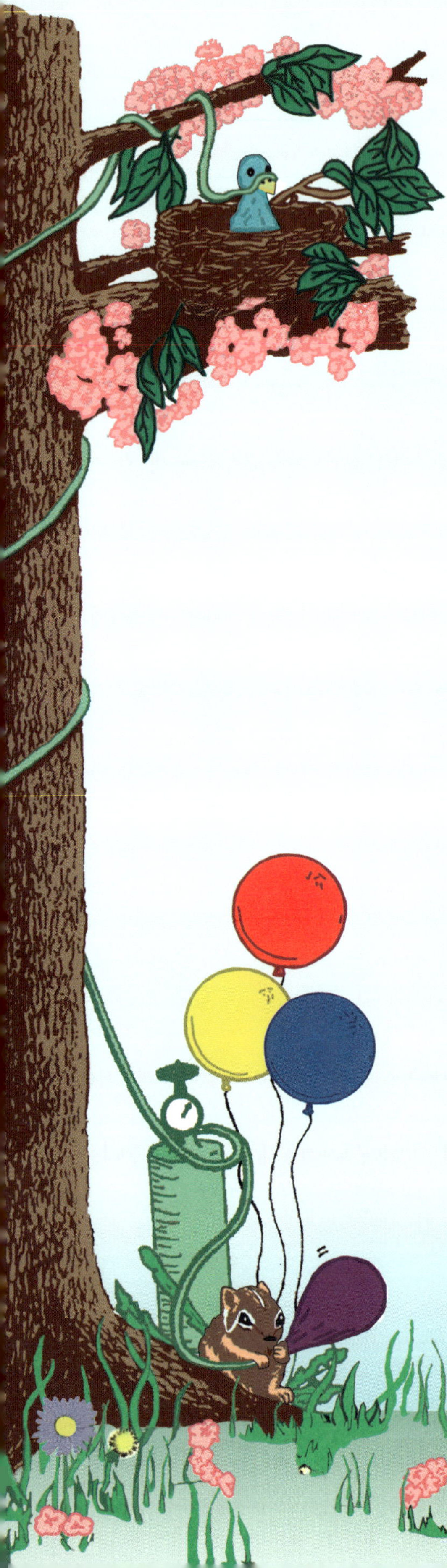

Ventilated

2-28-00 ______________   ______________
date started   *date stopped*

In an oxygen hood

______________   ______________
date started   *date stopped*

/ *On a nasal cannula*

______________   ______________
date started   *date stopped*

On ______________ *I was placed in room air.*
date

Your comments about my oxygen therapy

YOU WERE A VERY BAD BOY YOU COULD DO EVERYTHING BUT BREATHE. YOU TURNED BLUE IN YOUR MOTHERS ARMS

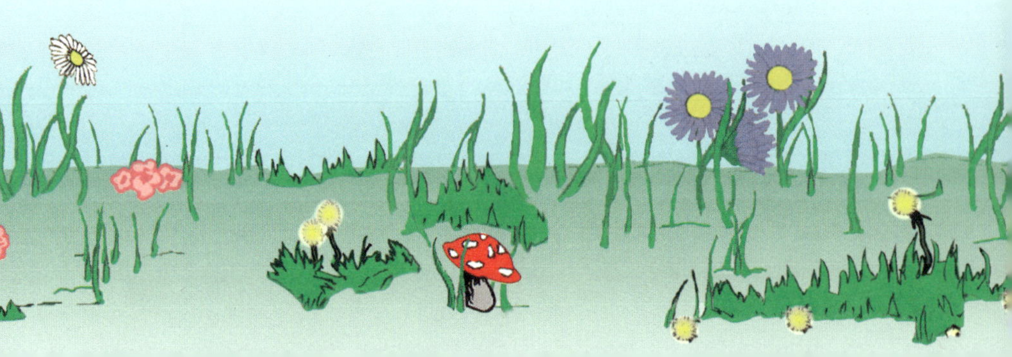

Baby's First Feedings

Because I was too little to eat, I was nourished with IVs. I had my IV for ________ days. On ________________

date

I was given my first gavage (tube) feeding. As I matured I was able to start nipple feedings.

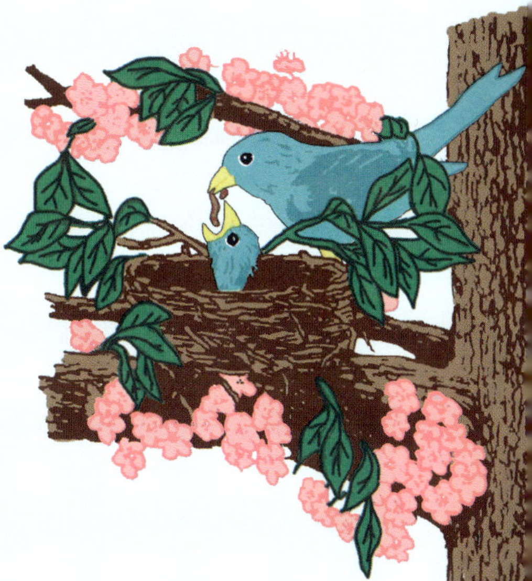

I first nursed from the bottle ________________ .

date

I was able to breast feed ________________ .

date

Mom fed me for the first time

Dad fed me for the first time

My Feeding Milestones

date	formula	amount	route	# hours between feedings

How old was I when I started sleeping all night?

Your comments about feedings

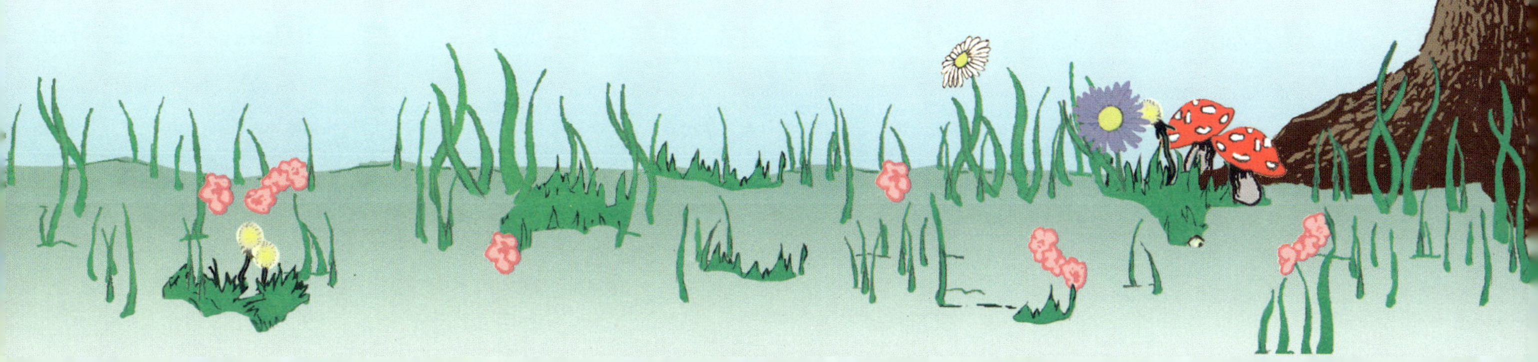

Special Procedures

Umbilical artery catheter (UAC) ______ ______

Umbilical venous catheter (UVC) ______ ______

Peripherally inserted central catheter (PICC) ______ ______

Chest tubes *right* *left* ______ ______

circle *date inserted* *date removed*

Phototherapy ______ ______

date started *date stopped*

X-Rays

Ultrasounds

date	*findings*

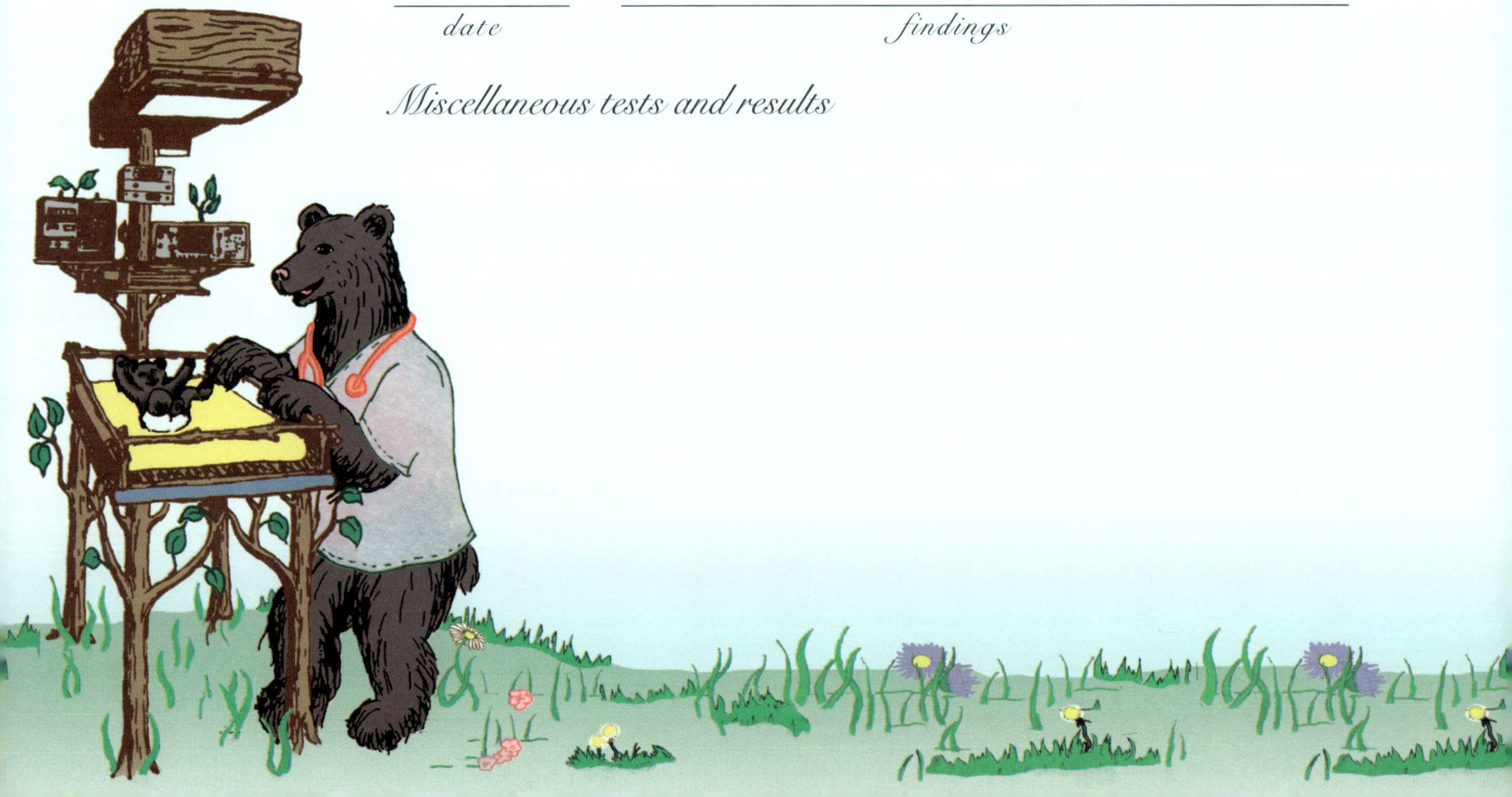

Miscellaneous tests and results

My blood type

Medications I received

name | *reason*

Transfusions I received

Eye examinations

date | *comments*

Surgeries

date | *surgeon* | *reason*

Your comments about my health status

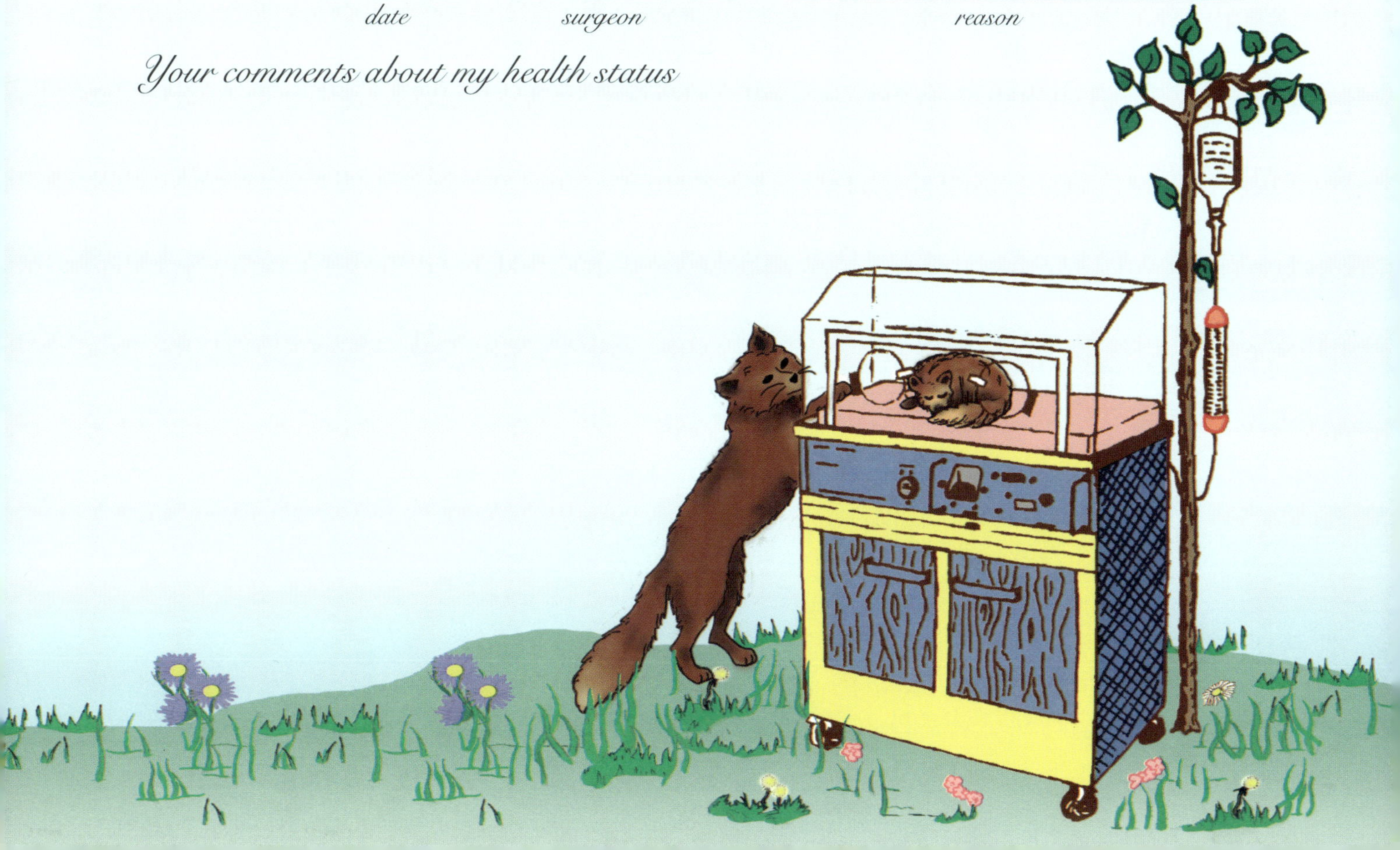

My Discharge Day

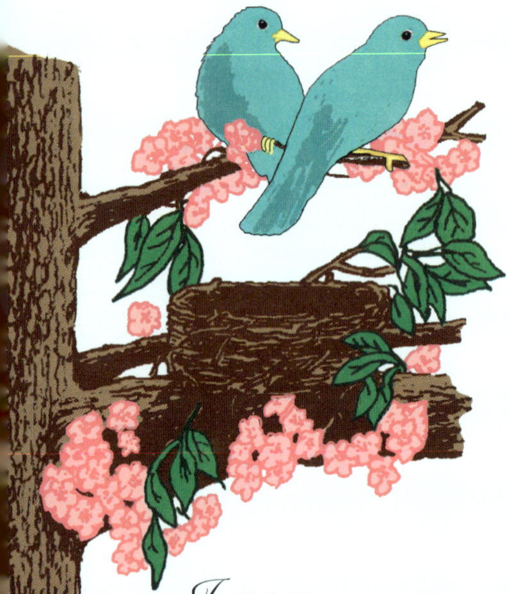

Date

Age

Weight

Length

I wore

Our address

To prepare for my homecoming you

What you forgot to bring

To celebrate we

Your comments

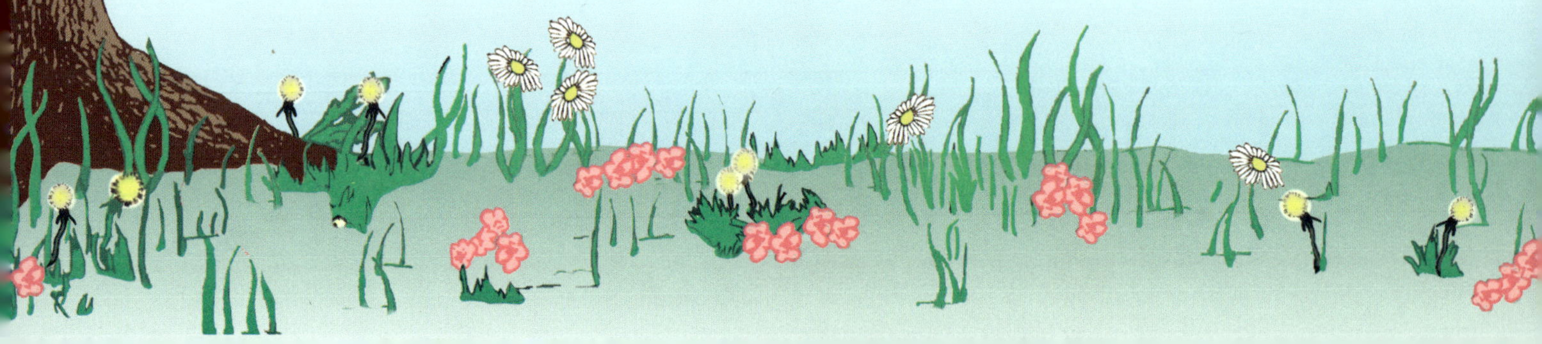

Comments and Autographs of My Doctors, Nurses and Visitors

My Birth Announcement

Gifts I Received

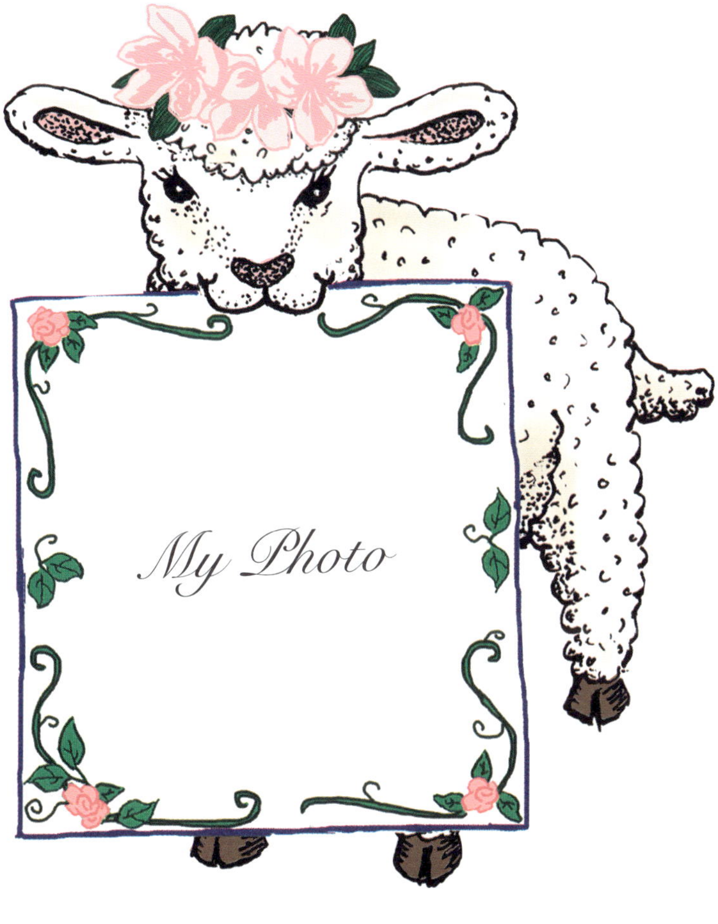
My Photo

I Was Just...

Held head up

Eye Contact

Took steps

Smiled

First tooth

Giggled

Cooed

Stood alone

Sat up

First word

Used potty

Crawled

. . . Amazing

Drank from a cup ______

Learned colors ______

First hair cut ______

First carnival ride ______

Snapped fingers ______

First airplane ride ______

Sang a song ______

Rode bicycle ______

Tied shoelaces ______

Dressed myself ______

Danced ______

Counted to ten ______

Tell Me About My Family

How old are you, Mommy? 25 *Daddy?* 39

Where was Mom born? SAN FRANCISCO CA. *Daddy?* VALLEJO CA

Were either of you premature? YES, DADDY

What schools did you attend?

What did you do the day I was born?
DADDY DROVE LIKE A MAD MAN TRYING TO GET TO THE HOSPITAL

What did you think the first time you saw me?
OH MY GOD LOOK HOW SMALL HE IS

Who do I look like? MOMMY SAYS HERE DADDY SAYS HI

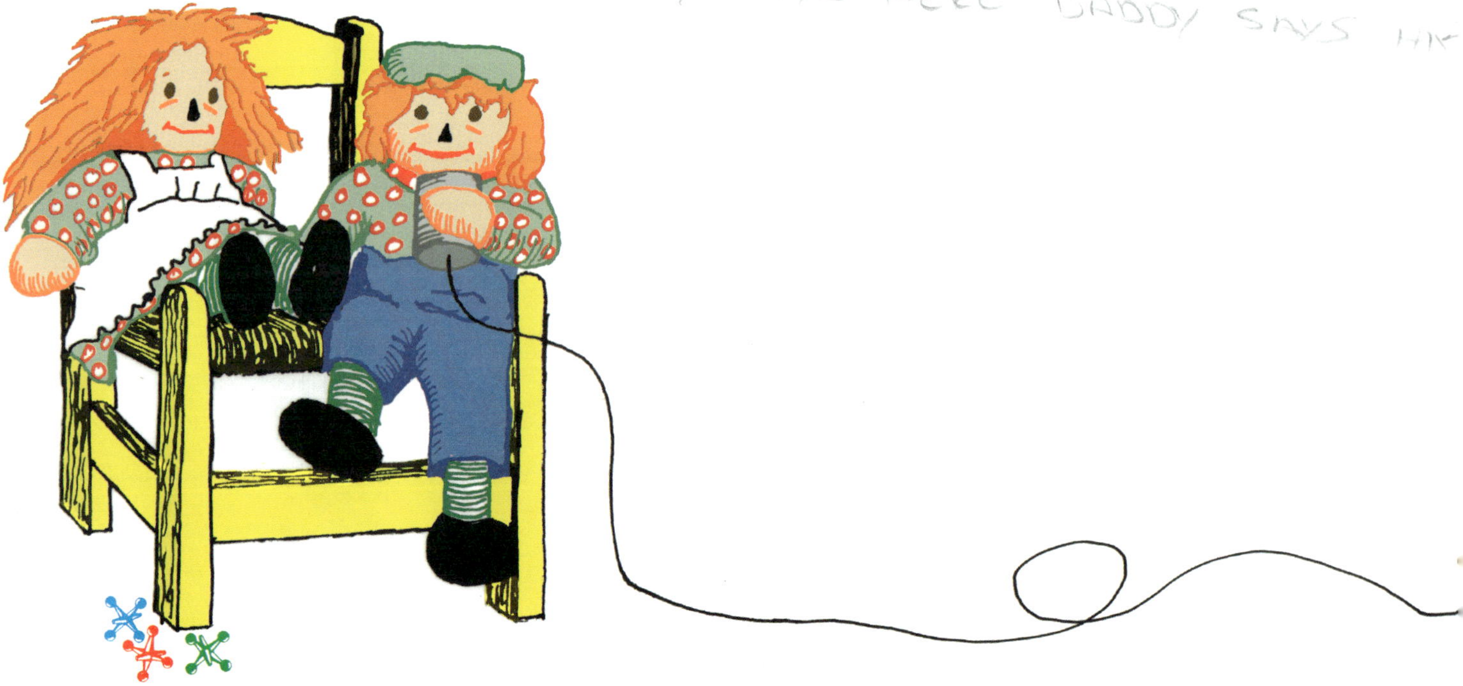

Do I have grandparents? YES

Do I have any brothers or sisters? YES

Who are my aunts and uncles?
Too many to write down.

Do I have cousins?
Yes, Josh, Austin, Adam, Tyler, Michelle & Chris

Who do I act like?
Mom & DAD

What did Mom look like while she was pregnant with me?
VERY PRETTY

picture

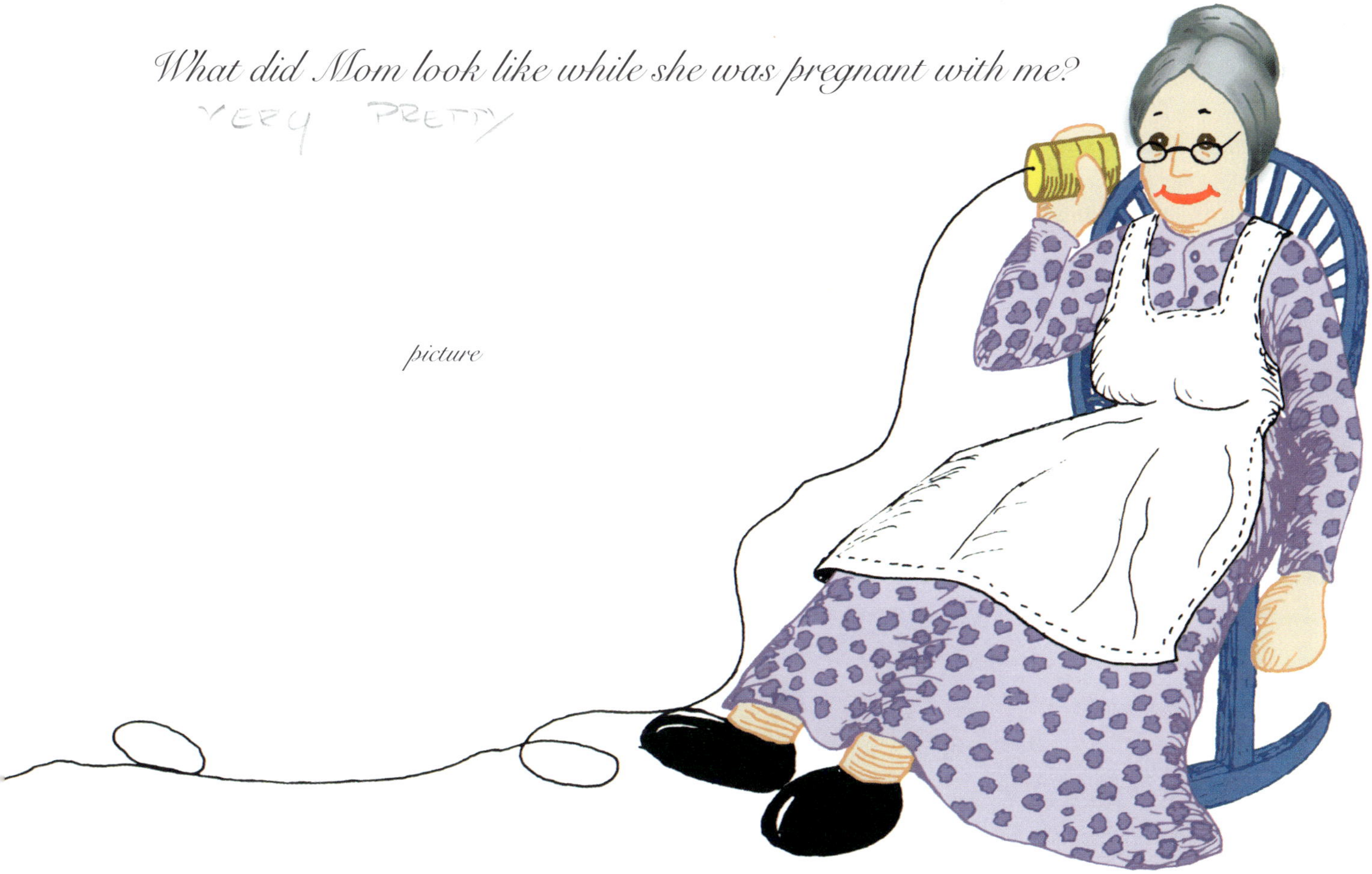

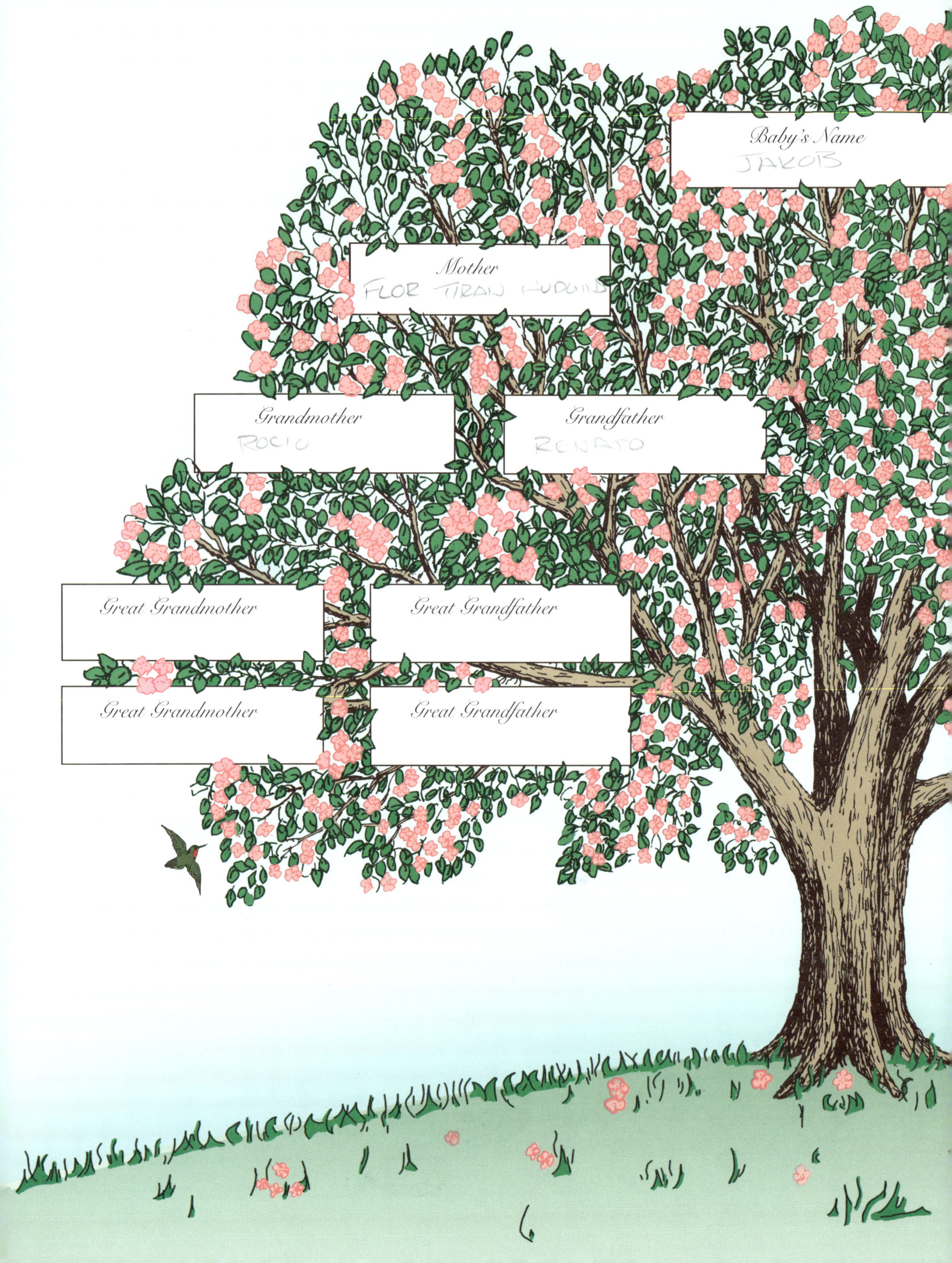

Baby's Name
JAKOB
Mother
FLOR TIRAN
Grandmother
ROCIO
Grandfather
RENATO
Great Grandmother
Great Grandfather
Great Grandmother
Great Grandfather

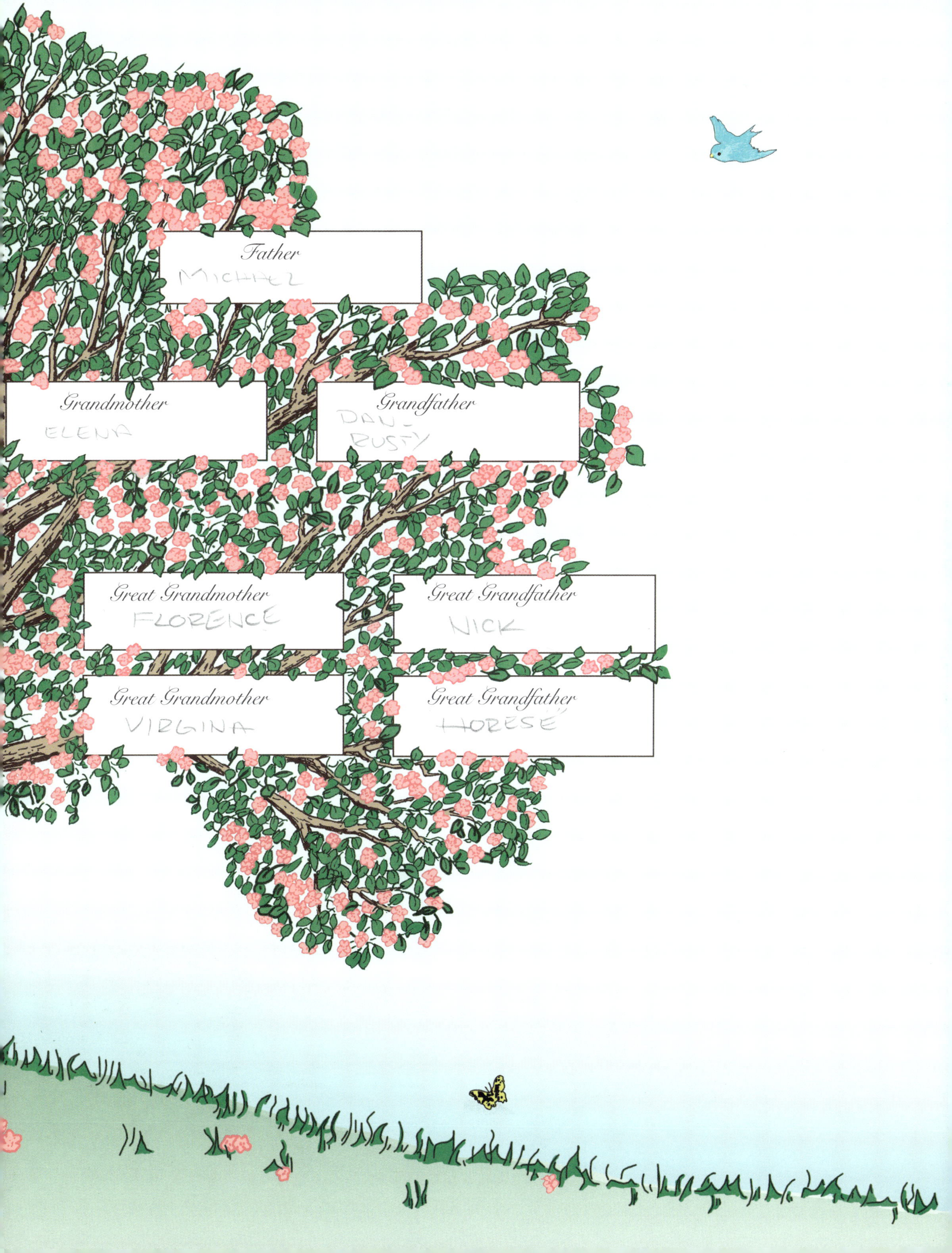

Father
MICHAEL
Grandmother
ELENA
Grandfather
DAN-
RUSTY
Great Grandmother
FLORENCE
Great Grandfather
NICK
Great Grandmother
VIRGINA
Great Grandfather
HORESE

My Daily Schedule

age

eating

sleeping

playing or favorite activity

age

eating

sleeping

playing or favorite activity

age

eating

sleeping

playing or favorite activity

age

eating

sleeping

playing or favorite activity

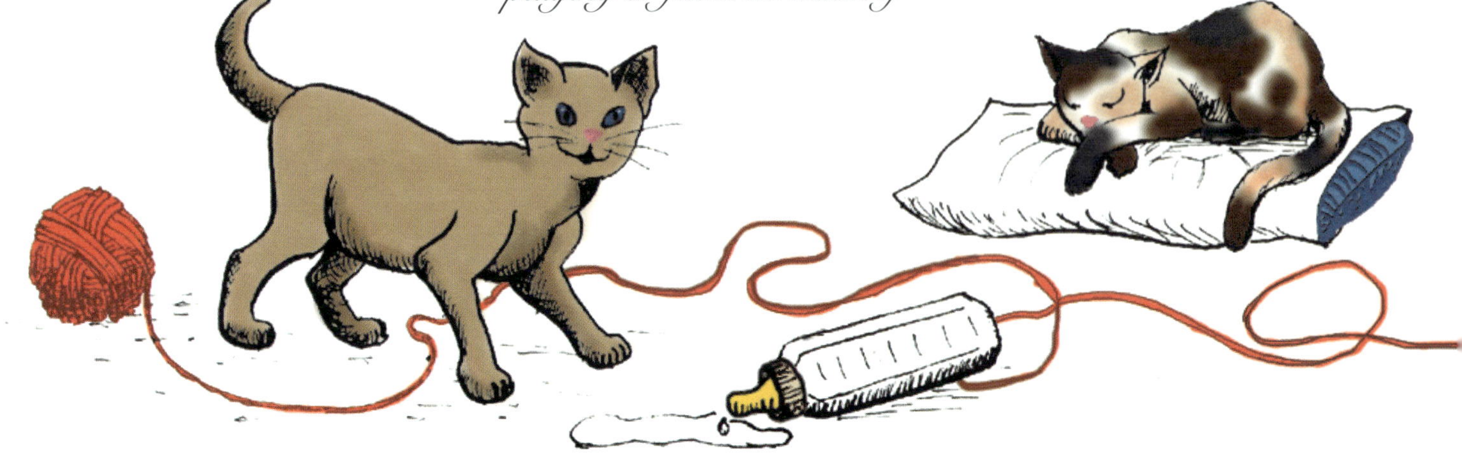

Suddenly I Grew

date	*weight*	*length*	*date*	*weight*	*length*

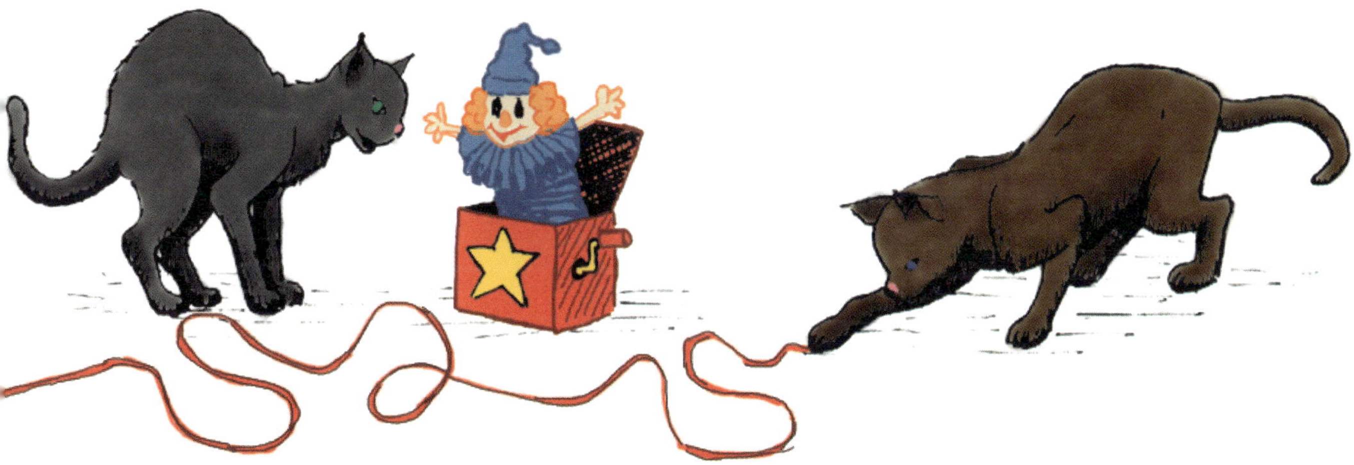

These Are a Few of My Favorite Things

my favorite food

phrase or rhyme

song

book or story

video

activity

game

toy

color

playmate

people

pet

dream and fantasy

Tell Me About My First Three Years

1

2

3

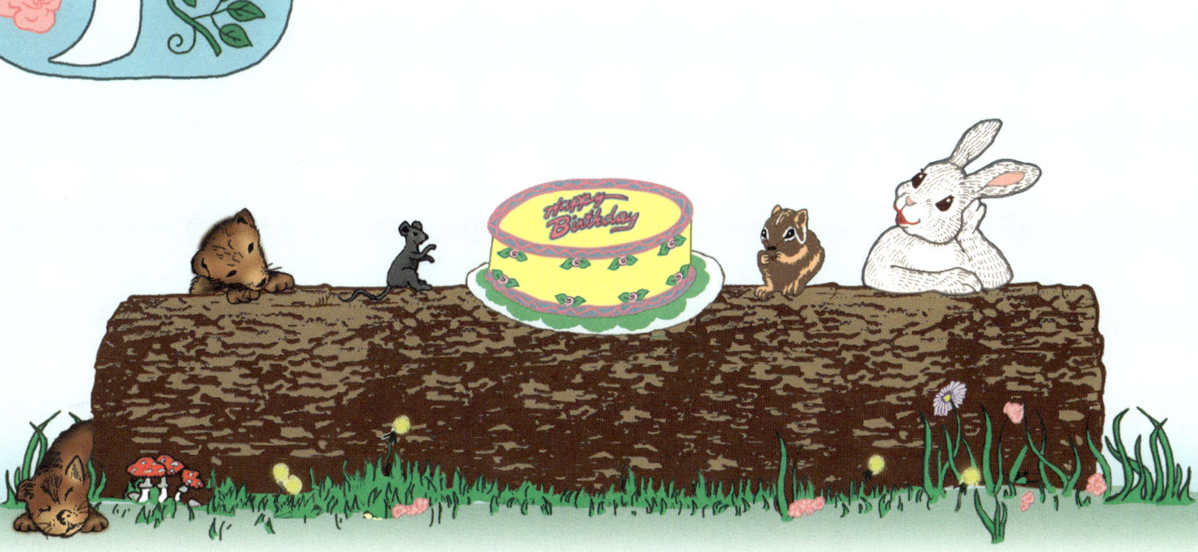

How Did I Change as I Grew and Got Ready for School?

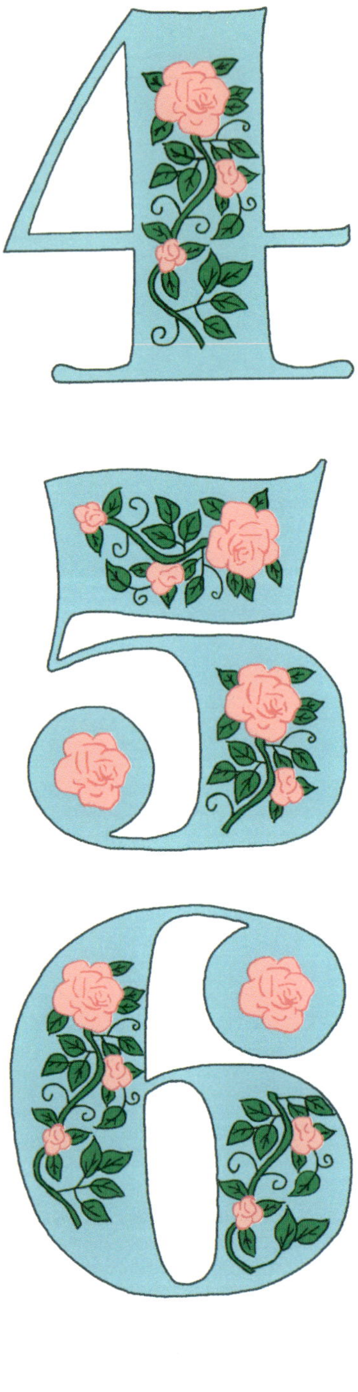

School Days

my photo

grade

teacher

best friend

my photo

grade

teacher

best friend

my photo

grade

teacher

best friend

my photo

grade

teacher

best friend

my photo

grade

teacher

best friend

my photo

grade

teacher

best friend

My first day of school

What I like most about school

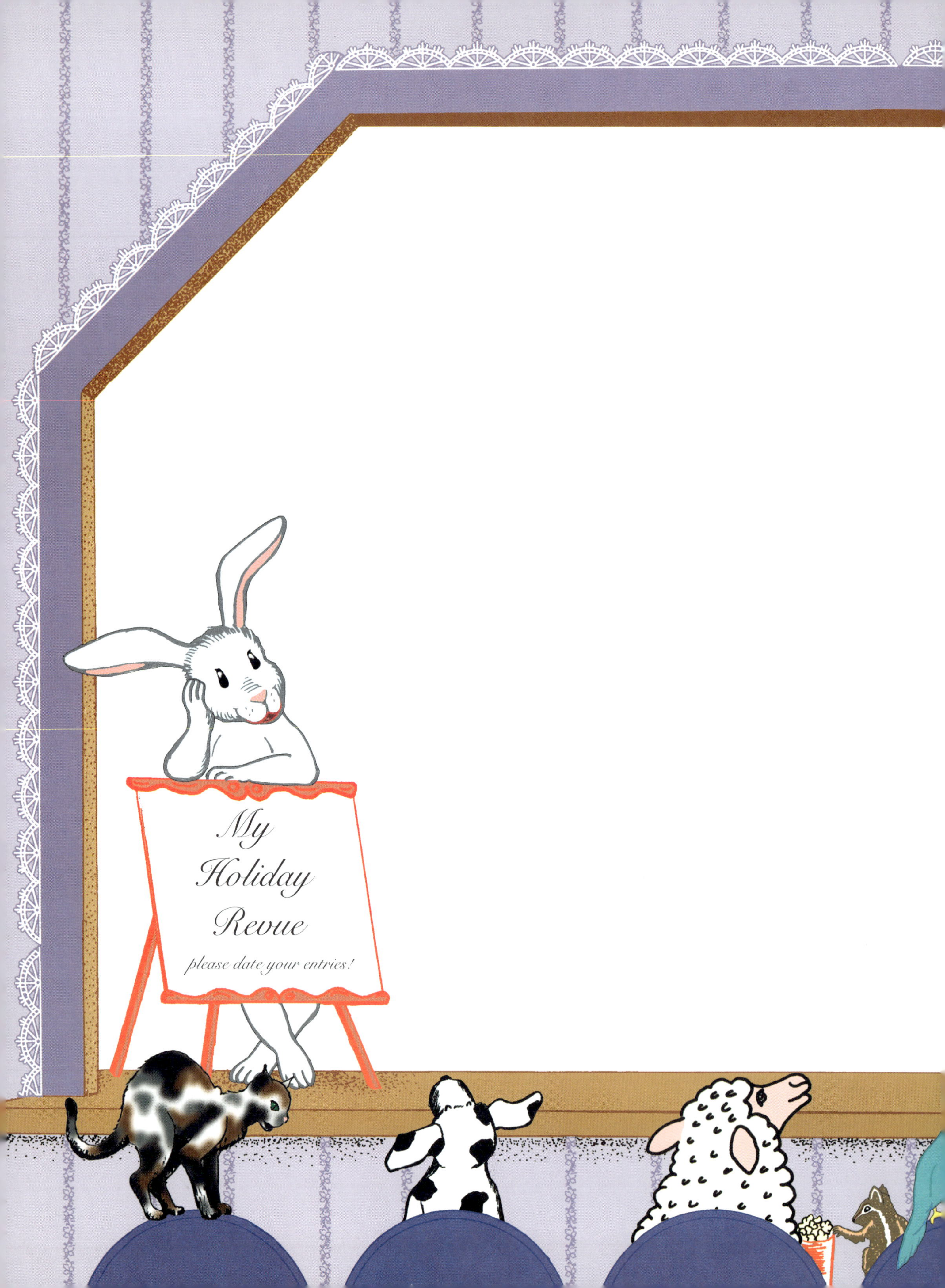
My
Holiday
Revue
please date your entries!

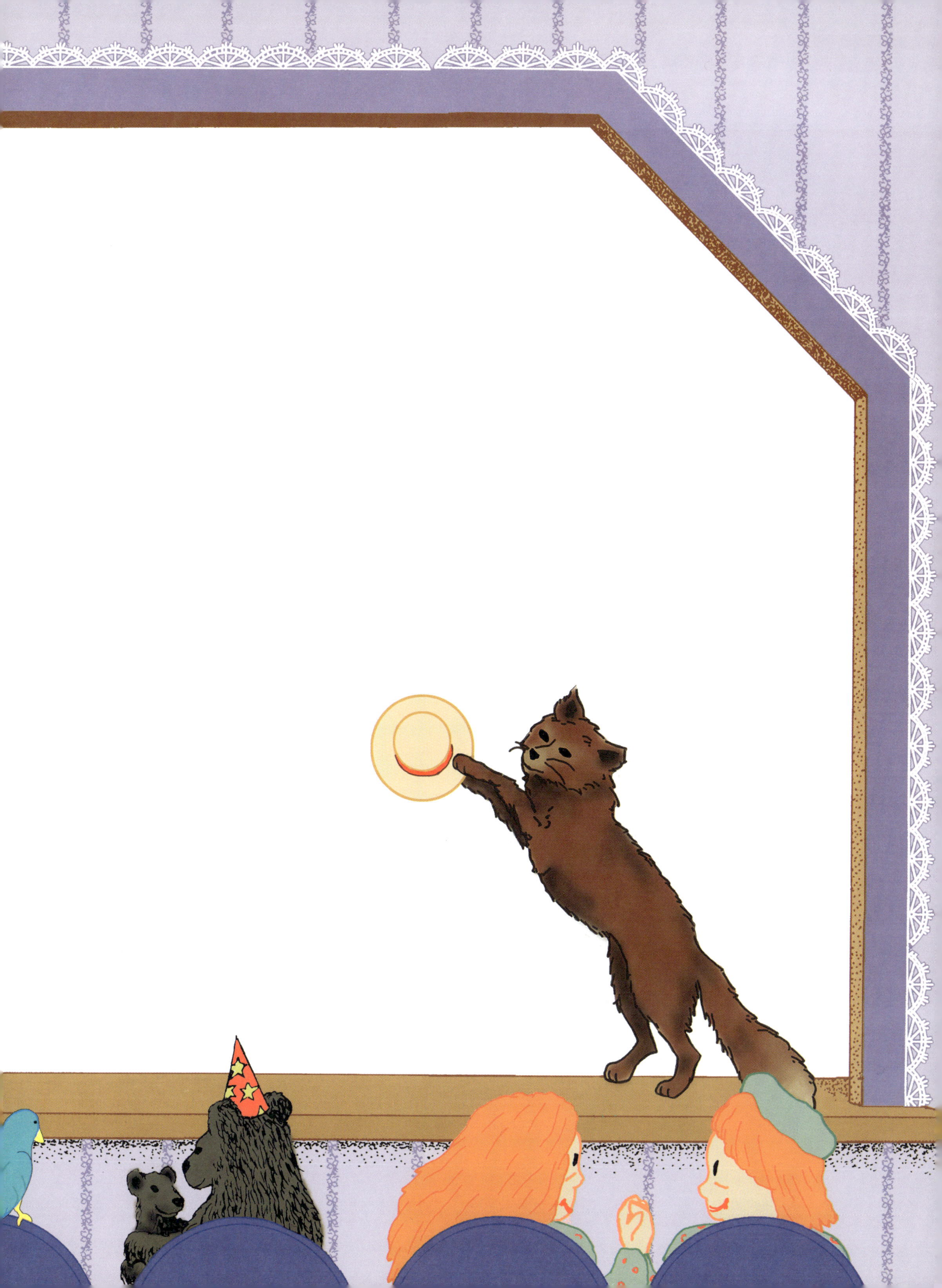

My Health Record

Immunizations	Birth	2 mo	4 mo	6 mo	12-15 mo	15-18 mo	4-6 yrs	11-12 yrs
DTP or DTaP		#1	#2	#3		#4	#5	Td
Polio		#1	#2		#3		#4	
Hib		#1	#2	#3	#4			
MMR					#1		#2	☆
Varicella					#1			☆
Hep B	#1	#2			#3			☆

Please date when I received my vaccinations

DTP: Diptheria, Tetanus, and Petussis Vaccine - Whole Cell
DTaP: Diptheria, Tetanus and Acellular Petusses Vaccine
Td: Tetanus and Diptheria Booster
Polio: Vaccine is given as OPV (Oral Polio Vaccine) or IPV (Inactivated Polio Vaccine)
Hib: Haemophilus Influenza Type B Vaccine
MMR: Measles, Mumps and Rubella Vaccine
Varicella: Chickenpox Vaccine
Hep B: Hepatitis B Vaccine

☆ Optional, depending on previous vaccine history.

Tests	*Date*	*Results*
Tuberculin		

Visits to the Doctor

My first visit

Other visits

My Dental Record

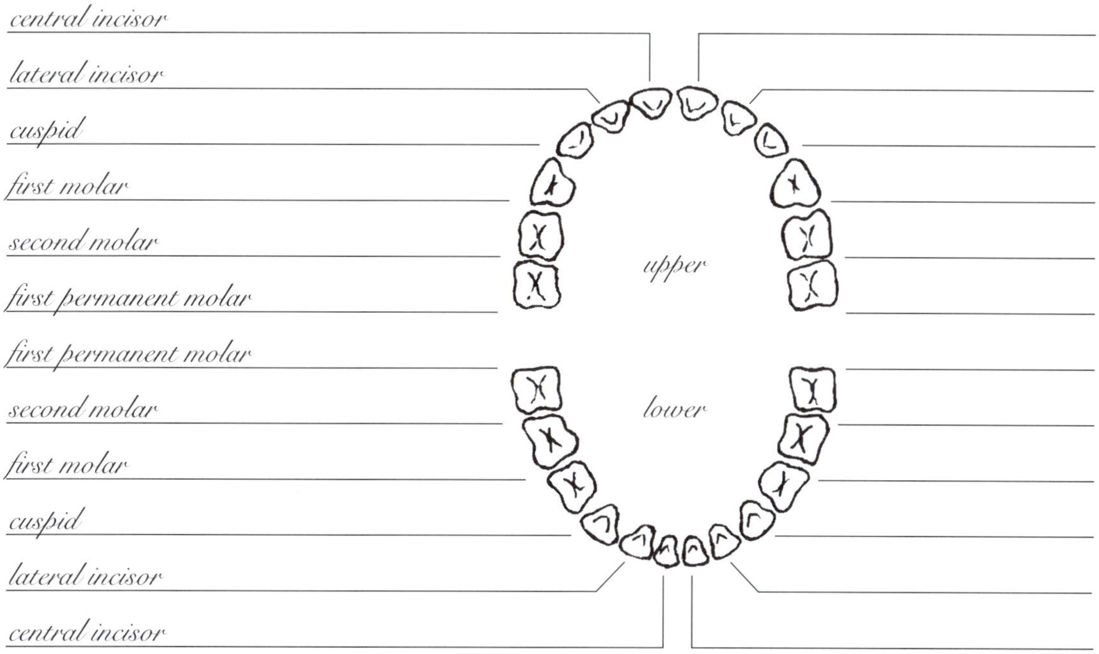

Please date when I got and lost my teeth.

Comments about my teething

I brushed my teeth by myself ____________________ .
date

Visits to the Dentist

My first visit

Other visitis

Baby's Journal

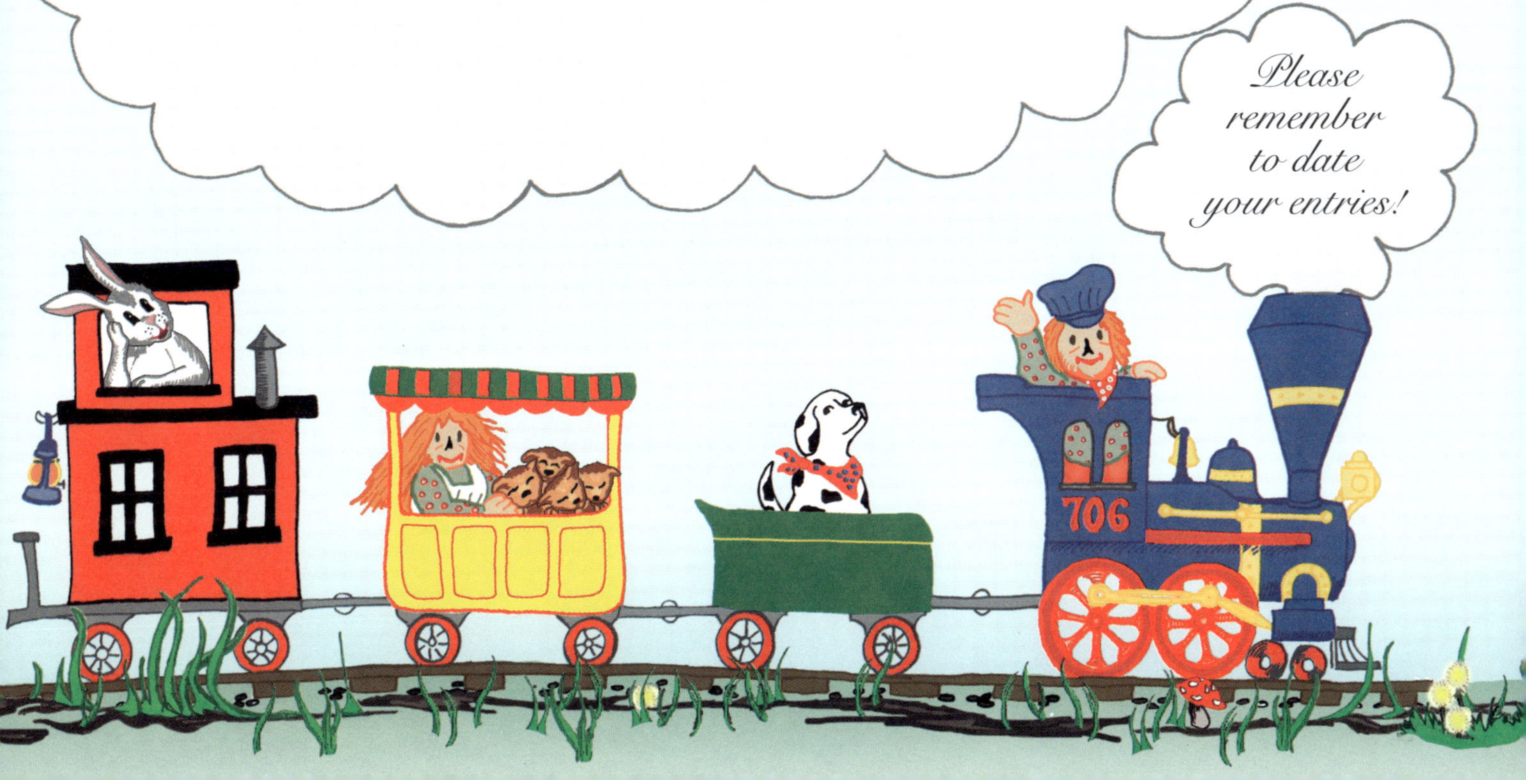
Please remember to date your entries!
706

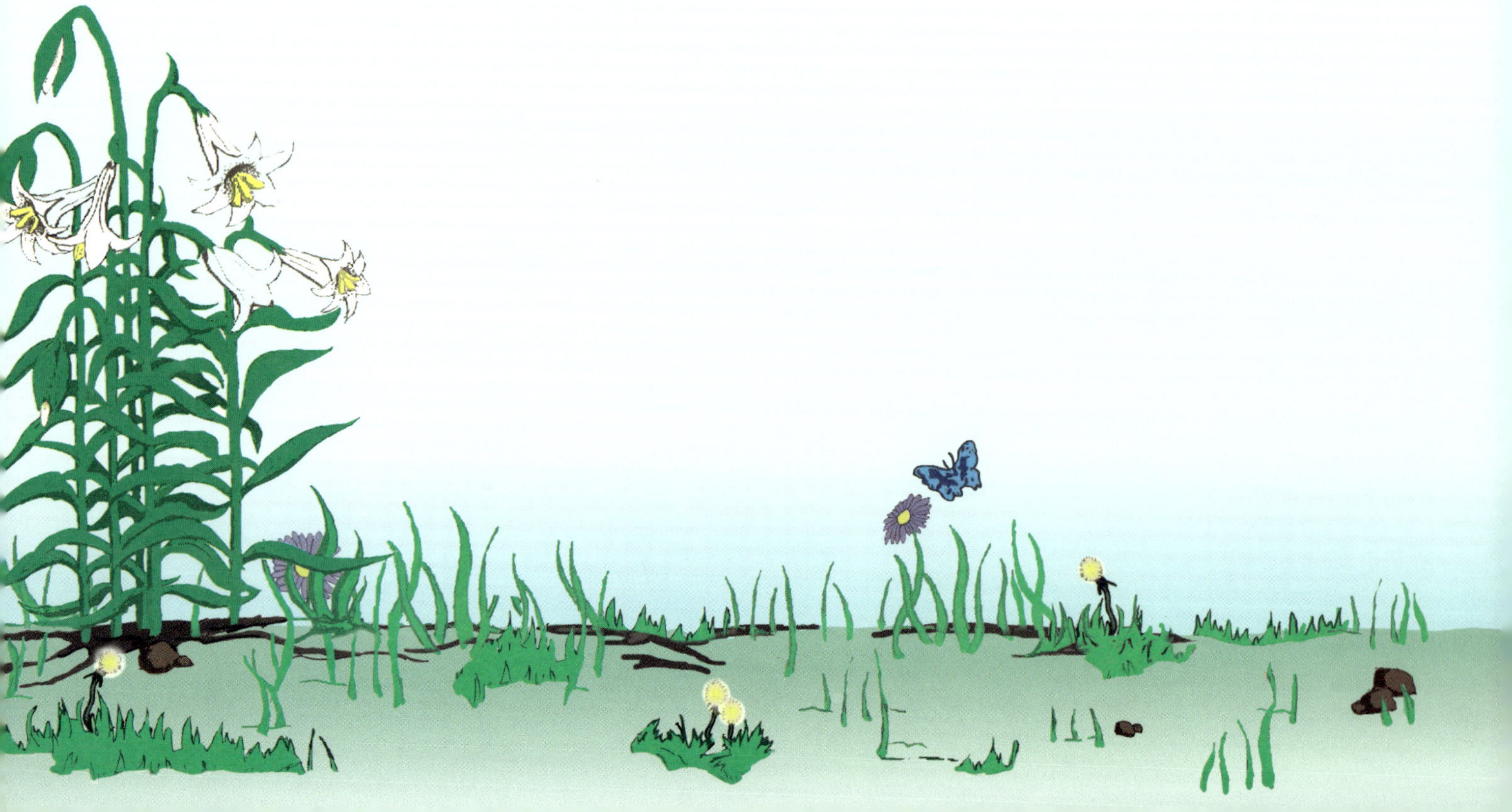

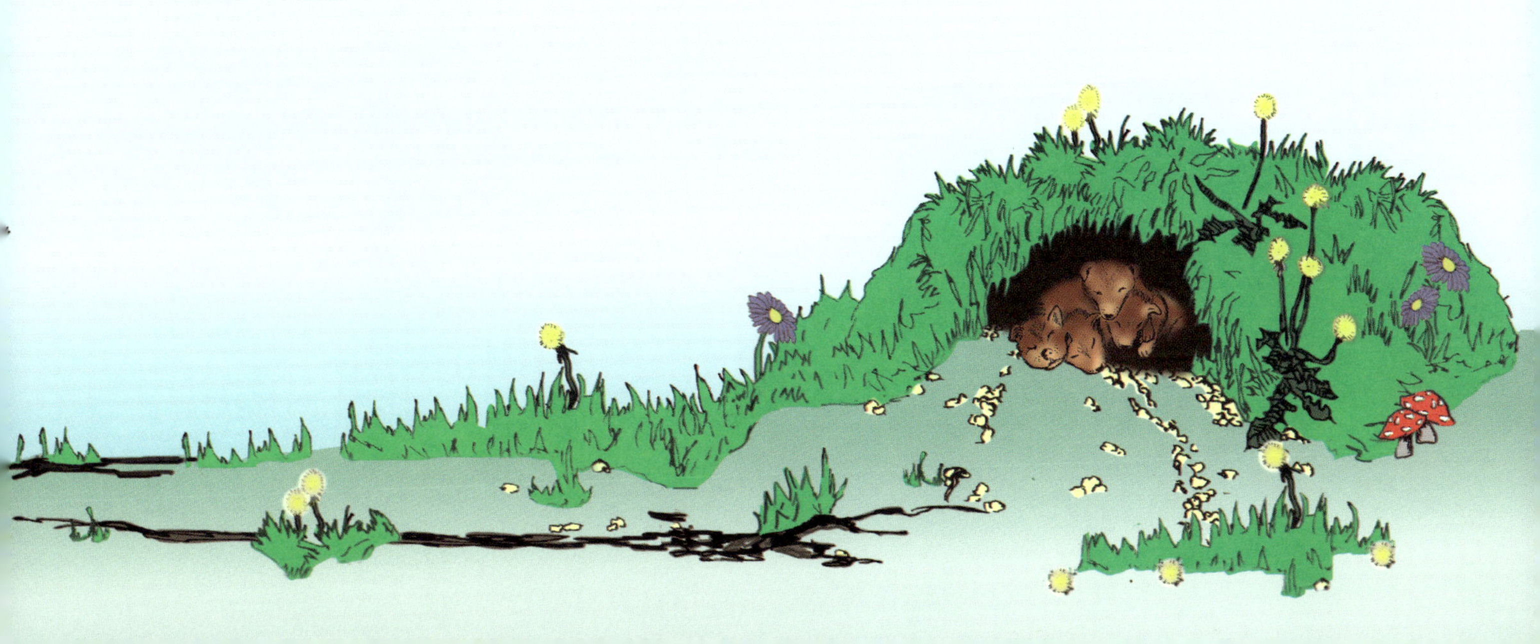

Precious Photographs

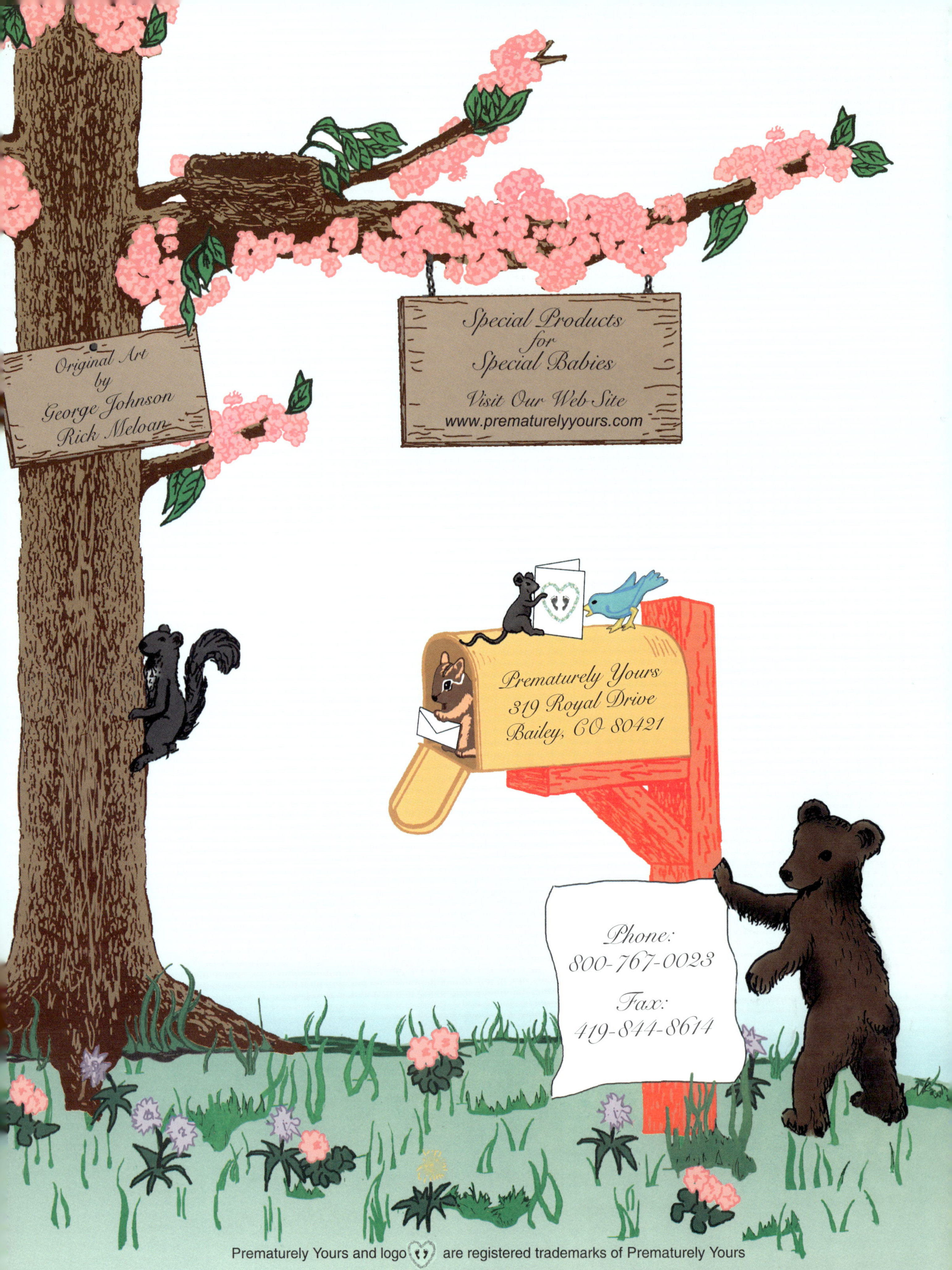
Original Art
by
George Johnson
Rick Meloan
Special Products
for
Special Babies
Visit Our Web-Site
www.prematurelyyours.com
Prematurely Yours
319 Royal Drive
Bailey, CO 80421
Phone:
800-767-0023
Fax:
419-844-8614